ASK DR. WEIL

YOUR TOP
HEALTH
CONCERNS

By Andrew Weil, M.D.:

Ask Dr. Weil
WOMEN'S HEALTH
YOUR TOP HEALTH CONCERNS
NATURAL REMEDIES
VITAMINS AND MINERALS
COMMON ILLNESSES
HEALTHY LIVING

8 WEEKS TO OPTIMUM HEALTH
SPONTANEOUS HEALING
NATURAL HEALTH, NATURAL MEDICINE
HEALTH AND HEALING
FROM CHOCOLATE TO MORPHINE
THE MARRIAGE OF THE SUN AND THE MOON
THE NATURAL MIND

ASK DR. WEIL

YOUR TOP HEALTH CONCERNS

Andrew Weil, M.D.

Edited by Steven Petrow

IVY BOOKS • NEW YORK

Ivy Books
Published by Ballantine Books
Copyright © 1997 by Great Bear Productions, LLC.

ISBN 0-8041-1677-6

Manufactured in the United States of America

Introduction

You've taken the first step toward optimum health. This book will give you more information about my philosophy along with answers to some of the questions I am asked most frequently.

I wrote *Spontaneous Healing* and *8 Weeks to Optimum Health* because I wanted to call attention to the innate, intrinsic nature of the healing process. I've always believed that the body can heal itself if you give it a chance. Why? Because it has a healing system. If you're feeling well, it's important to know about this system so that you can enhance your well-being. If you are ill, you'll also want to know about it because it is your best hope of recovery.

To maintain optimum health requires commitment. This book—and the others in the series—can give you much of the basic information you need about diet, supplements, common illnesses, natural remedies, and healthy living.

All of these questions originated on "Ask Dr. Weil," my program on the World Wide Web. If you still have questions, come visit the clinic at www.drweil.com.

What's in Your Antioxidant Cocktail?

Q:
What vitamins should I be taking on a regular basis?

A:
I get asked about the antioxidant "cocktail" perhaps more than about any other subject. You can really help your body by taking protective antioxidants, nutrients that protect tissues by blocking the chemical reactions by which many toxins cause harm. One way to go about it is to increase your consumption of fresh fruits and vegetables. You can also take supplements.

Here is the formula I use myself and recommend to my patients:

- *Vitamin C:* 1,000 to 2,000 milligrams two to three times a day. Your body can absorb this vitamin more easily in a soluble powder form than in a large tablet. I take a dose of vitamin C with breakfast and dinner, and, if I can remember, another before bed. Plain ascorbic acid may irritate a sensitive stomach, so take it with food or look for a buffered or nonacidic form.
- *Vitamin E:* 400 to 800 IU a day. People under forty should take 400 IU a day; people over forty, 800 IU. Since vitamin E is fat soluble, it must be taken with food to be absorbed. Also, natural vitamin E (d-alpha-tocopherol) is much better than the synthetic form (dl-alpha-tocopherol). I usually take vitamin E at lunch. Make sure the product contains the other tocopherols,

especially gamma, which offers protection that alpha-tocopherol does not.

- *Selenium:* 200 to 300 micrograms a day. Selenium is a trace mineral with antioxidant and anticancer properties. Selenium and vitamin E facilitate each other's absorption, so take them together. Vitamin C may interfere with the absorption of some forms of selenium, so take them separately. Doses above 400 micrograms a day may not be healthy.

- *Mixed carotenes:* 25,000 IU a day. I take mixed carotenes as a supplement with my breakfast. I recommend a natural form—easily found in health food stores. Men: read the label to make sure it gives you lycopene, the red pigment in tomatoes that helps prevent prostate cancer.

All in all, this is a simple formula that will not cost you too much trouble or money.

Is Aspartame Dangerous?

Q:
I think I've had an adverse reaction to aspartame. I've used NutraSweet for fifteen years, usually consuming six to eight packets a day. Now I have reduced motor control of my arms and hands. Is there a link? What do you recommend?

A:
First of all, I would stop using NutraSweet. The manufacturer portrays aspartame as a gift from nature, but although the two component parts do occur naturally, aspartame itself does not. Like all artificial sweeteners, aspartame has a peculiar taste. Because I have seen a number of patients—mostly women—who report headaches from using it, I don't view it as nontoxic or biologically inert. Some women also find that aspartame aggravates PMS. There are no proven long-term side effects, but there's a lot of suspicion.

In general, I think you're better off using moderate amounts of sugar. People who use NutraSweet to control their weight should know there's not a shred of evidence that the availability or use of artificial sweeteners has helped anyone to lose weight. Think about it: You have pie à la mode for dessert (about 495 calories), and then you use a packet of NutraSweet for your coffee (saving 18 calories). There's something wrong with that calculation. Also, remember that aspartame turns up in unexpected items. Recently, on an airplane, I was given some

3

mints that were sweetened with aspartame. Most people wouldn't have noticed this.

As for your motor troubles, I would advise going to a neurologist for an evaluation. Your condition may be unrelated to aspartame, although there is some anecdotal evidence indicating a link.

Treatment for Athlete's Foot?

Q:
My feet are itchy. Is grapefruit seed extract really as good for athlete's foot as the guy at the health food store claims?

A:
Athlete's foot is a fungal infection of the skin, related to jock itch and ringworm. As you probably know, it thrives in moist, warm, dark places, so one of the best treatments I can recommend is exposing your feet to fresh air and sunlight. Keep them clean and dry—and wear sandals if you can.

I've also heard a lot of positive testimonials about grapefruit seed extract, which is available at health food stores. It is reported to have significant antifungal effects. Apply the extract (full strength) two to three times a day to the affected area.

Tea tree oil, extracted from the leaves of *Melaleuca alternifolia*, a tree native to Australia, is another home remedy that works as well as or better than over-the-counter medications like Tinactin and Lotrimin. Apply a light coating of this product to the affected area three or four times a day, and continue to apply it for two weeks after the infection seems to have disappeared. You want to make sure the fungus is eradicated. Tea tree oil will also clear up fungal infections of the toenails or finger-nails, conditions that are usually difficult to cure, even with strong systemic antibiotics. It's also effective for

ringworm and jock itch as well as bacterial infections of
the skin. You'll find tea tree oil products at health food
and herb stores. Be sure to select ones that are 100 percent tea tree oil.

Do B-12 Boosters Work?

Q:

What do you think of taking B-12 to boost energy? Some friends of mine get shots regularly and say the vitamin works wonders.

A:

B-12 works in the body by helping the bone marrow regenerate red blood cells. The vitamin has been linked to protection against heart disease, and against mental deterioration such as memory loss. People use it to boost their energy, to recuperate from frequent partying with alcohol, and to revitalize themselves during menstruation.

Many people take vitamin B-12 shots as a quick way to pump up their energy level. I see this particularly among entertainers and theater people before performances. But most of them aren't deficient in B-12, so the shots are acting as very effective placebos. A placebo is a medicine or drug that doesn't have any direct chemical effect, but because of belief in its effectiveness, the patient experiences benefit. Placebo responses can be extremely powerful, and B-12 shots can definitely elicit them.

Most people I know who get B-12 shots say the first one filled them with a warm glow and a flush of energy. They felt terrific. But subsequent injections don't usually measure up. That's typical of placebos. Extreme fatigue, however, can be a symptom of B-12 deficiency, but that needs to be confirmed by blood tests.

People take B-12 in the form of shots because it's not

always easily absorbed through the stomach, and it needs to be combined with calcium to be useful to the body. So injections are the most effective way to get it into your system. If you hate shots, you can take the vitamin as a nasal spray, a nasal gel, or a lozenge you put under your tongue. You can also get it in a time-release formula combined with sorbitol for better absorption through the small intestine.

It's not hard to get enough B-12 in an ordinary diet. The body gets this vitamin almost exclusively from animal sources, such as liver, pork, milk, and eggs. Vegetarians, especially vegans, are at risk for deficiency, especially vegan children. Many older people have trouble absorbing the vitamin from foods. B-12 deficiency results in pernicious anemia, which can produce such symptoms as weakness, apathy, light-headedness, shortness of breath, numbness in the extremities, and loss of balance. There may also be accompanying psychiatric changes such as paranoia and depression. In the elderly, B-12 deficiency can cause memory loss and disorientation that may be confused with Alzheimer's disease. All these symptoms can usually be reversed with supplemental B-12.

Experiment as you wish. B-12 is effective in very small doses, but has been found to be harmless even in amounts much higher than the 6 micrograms recommended daily.

Plagued by an Aching Back?

Q:
What do I do for lower back pain?

A:
Chronic back pain is often caused by unbalanced nervous control of the musculature, which triggers muscle contraction, reduction of normal blood supply, and inflammation. In most cases, it's not directly caused by structural injury, although injury can create a focal point for the effects of neuromuscular imbalance.

What you're feeling is the end result of a chain of nervous system events that starts in your brain and leads to pain in your back. Because the nervous system is connected to the mind and the emotions, healing is best directed there, often the root of the trouble. This isn't to say that your pain is all in your head, but rather that the vicious cycle of muscle spasm may have an emotional basis. John Sarno, M.D., calls most cases of chronic back pain "tension myositis syndrome," referring to psychosomatic inflammation of the muscles. He has a great book on the subject called *Healing Back Pain*.

So rather than looking to chiropractors, osteopaths, acupuncturists, or massage practitioners to cure the pain, I'd try to understand the real nature of the problem and consider mental and emotional changes. Sometimes it may do the trick just to understand that the pain can depart once your brain stops sending the wrong messages to your back. Think about restructuring the patterns of

9

thinking, feeling, and managing stress that lead your nervous system to spasm.

You can take steps to strengthen your back and improve the health of the muscles that contribute to the pain. Yoga is a wonderful way to improve flexibility and balance your nervous system. Stretches that target your hamstrings are a good way to make sure your back gets the support it needs. Abdominal strengthening exercises will also help.

The way you sit is important, too, especially if you spend long days at a computer or a desk. Sit a bit forward on your chair, with your knees comfortably apart and heels on the floor, your pelvis rotated slightly forward with your body balanced on top. If you place a rolled-up towel under your tailbone, it will help you achieve a good sitting posture. Don't puff out your chest; that's hard on your back, too.

There may also be a link between back pain and diet. One study found that arteries narrowed by atherosclerosis—avoidable with a low-fat diet—can't deliver as much blood to the lower back, and this affects disks, muscles, and nerves.

If you have an episode of acute lower back pain, use ice on the area as soon as you can. Chiropractic manipulation has also been shown to help. And keep in mind that almost everyone who suffers from acute back pain recovers in about a month with or without treatment.

Betting or Bailing on Beta-Carotene?

Q:
I've started to take 20,000 IU of beta-carotene a day per your suggestion. Recently I have read that beta-carotene supplements, even in these modest quantities, can be toxic. What is your latest opinion on the subject?

A:
Beta-carotene is not toxic, and there are no studies that suggest it may be. We do have some new information on the supplement, however, that shows it's not the panacea some people had hoped.

The interest in beta-carotene went mainstream after about two dozen studies showed that people with lots of beta-carotene-rich fruits and vegetables in their diets got less cancer and heart disease. As one of the vitamins that neutralize "free radical" molecules in the body, beta-carotene seemed to make sense as a preventive to oxidative damage leading to cancer.

But the results of giving the vitamin as a supplement were not all encouraging. A Finnish study reported 18 percent more cases of lung cancer among heavy smokers who took beta-carotene supplements. Then, National Cancer Institute researchers halted a study on the effects of beta-carotene and vitamin A. Smokers taking the supplements had 28 percent more instances of lung cancer than those taking the placebo.

And a twelve-year study of 22,000 physicians found

no evidence that beta-carotene supplements were protective against cancer and heart disease.

It's important to note that none of these studies showed that beta-carotene caused cancer. They weren't designed to ask that question. But they do indicate that beta-carotene fails to prevent cancer among smokers. No one is certain why. Some researchers point out that antioxidants can promote free radicals under certain circumstances, rather than keeping them under control—and perhaps smoking triggers this action.

It's likely that cancer was already established in the men who were diagnosed with it during these trials. No one believes that antioxidants can cure existing cancers. But study after study has shown the protective effect of high levels of beta-carotene in the blood—and of large amounts of fruits and vegetables in the diet. It is probably not beta-carotene alone that is responsible. It could be the whole family of carotenoid pigments. (And so far, we don't have findings on the effects of beta-carotene in women. The Women's Antioxidant and Cardiovascular Study is continuing despite the negative findings in men.)

We know of about five hundred carotenoids, the family of substances that the body converts into vitamin A. I recommend taking advantage of them all. Eat a diet rich in fruits and vegetables, especially peaches, melons, mangoes, sweet potatoes, squash, pumpkins, tomatoes, and dark leafy greens. And if you cannot include enough of these in your diet, you may want to take a supplement. I recommend a mixed carotene supplement. Take one capsule (25,000 IU) a day. Inquire in a health food store about these new products.

Does Blue-Green Algae Boost Energy?

Q:
I'm curious about the blue-green algae thing. I was a total disbeliever in the high energy and healing claims many people reported to me, but I was worn down by friends and started taking it. It worked! What do you know and think about this?

A:
Frankly, I don't have any firsthand experience with blue-green algae. Like you, I've heard testimonials from people about its energy-boosting effects. According to what I've read, there is very little research on the chemistry or pharmacology of blue-green algae, but I found one unsettling paper indicating that the species used for commercial purposes is capable of producing liver and nerve toxins, which could be unhealthy in long-term use. Many users report druglike stimulation from these products. Until I know what's responsible for that effect, I'm not going to recommend them. I've seen dozens of sites on the Web and many print advertisements promoting blue-green algae as a wonder food and an incredible business opportunity. Caveat emptor. Overall, I'd say wait and see on this. If it works for you, use it, but keep your eye out for new information.

If low energy is a problem for you, you could consider using ginseng, a natural tonic. Used on a regular basis, ginseng increases energy, vitality, and sexual vigor, and provides resistance to all kinds of stress. It is nontoxic, but Asian ginseng (*Panax ginseng*) can raise blood pressure and is more of a stimulant. I often recommend American ginseng (*Panax quinquefolius*) to people who are chronically ill and to those lacking in vitality.

Crippled by Carpal Tunnel Syndrome?

Q:
Due to repetitive typing I have developed carpal tunnel syndrome in both arms. I was given anti-inflammatory medication for this. Then I developed stomach problems—gastritis and irritable bowel syndrome. After two years of getting all kinds of tests done and having doctors tell me that I was going to have to live with this the rest of my life, I got fed up. I recently have begun to see a doctor of Eastern medicine, who started me on herbs including ginger tablets with DGL (deglycyrrhizinated licorice). On my second visit he performed acupuncture. I have started to feel better. Do you think that with Eastern medicine my carpal tunnel will also get better?

A:
When you're an especially speedy typist or spend long hours at the keyboard, the tendons that move the fingers can swell. There's one little tunnel of ligamentous tissue at the base of your palm that all the tendons and one very important nerve pass through from your arm to your hand. That's where the swelling and pressure can become especially painful and irritating, causing a condition known as carpal tunnel syndrome (CTS).

The most effective treatment that I've found is vitamin B-6 (pyridoxine), 100 milligrams, two or three times a day. In this dosage, pyridoxine is not acting as a B vitamin but rather as a natural therapeutic agent that relieves nerve compression injuries. Be aware that doses of B-6 higher than 300 milligrams a day have caused rare cases of nerve damage. Discontinue usage if you develop any unusual numbness. (A much-publicized University of Michigan study warned about nerve toxicity with B-6 and discouraged people from using it for CTS. I disagree.)

For quick relief when you're hurting, rub on arnica gel, which you can find in your health food store or drugstore. Also, try wrapping ice packs around your wrists (a bag of frozen peas works just as well); if you use this treatment for five minutes every few hours when you're especially stressing your wrists, it may ease the pain and the inflammation. The ginger you mention may relieve inflammation, and acupuncture certainly can provide symptomatic relief.

The most important consideration when you've got CTS is to figure out ways to reduce your typing. Unless you reduce the strain on your wrists, long-term improvement is unlikely. That means less typing, and learning how to stop driving yourself so hard at the keyboard. There are a couple of other things you can try. Make yourself stand up every hour for a few minutes and stretch. The muscles in your wrists are connected all the way up through your arms, across your shoulders, and up into your neck. Pay attention to those parts of your body, too, because stretching and relaxing your shoulders, neck, and back can ease the strain on your wrists. I know some people who've found a lot of relief through deep-tissue massage or Rolfing. And consider whether you're feeling some emotional tension at work that tightens your whole body, making it more susceptible to injury.

Your posture at the keyboard can make a big difference. Sit up straight, with your weight slightly forward. Your feet should be flat on the floor, or tilted comfortably on an adjustable footrest. An adjustable keyboard tray allows you to change the position of your hands now and then, and helps you keep your wrists straight, with your forearms horizontal and at a 90-degree angle to your upper arms. Your elbows should be at your sides in a relaxed position. Every now and then, tilt your head slowly to each side, and roll your shoulders twice forward and twice back. Squeeze your hands into tight fists and then stretch your fingers out as wide as they will go. Close your hands into fists again and rotate your wrists a few times in either direction.

Help for Chronic
Fatigue Syndrome?

Q:
*My wife has had chronic fatigue syndrome for the past
six years. Traditional medicine has seemed to offer very
little to her and in the past has actually made her worse.
Many M.D.s, including many who specialize in the field,
still seem not to have a clue about how to treat this illness. What suggestions do you have for overcoming this
disease?*

A:
Many people have written in about chronic fatigue syndrome (CFS), a condition known incorrectly as "chronic
Epstein-Barr virus disease" or "chronic EBV." I'm not
sure anybody knows exactly what chronic fatigue syndrome is; right now it appears to be a faddish disease that
may or may not prove to be a true clinical entity. My suspicion is that if you look at a hundred people with the diagnosis, you might actually find many different conditions
present—some purely emotional (such as depression) and
others that might involve chronic viral infections.

The most important information I can give you is that
the syndrome will end. Don't believe people who tell you
otherwise.

I agree that conventional medicine has little to offer.
Some doctors attempt treatment with injections of
gamma globulin, interferon, or the antiviral drug acyclovir. These are pretty drastic methods that may do more
harm than good. It sounds as though your wife has al-

ready been subjected to some of these treatments; generally I advise staying away from them.

Unfortunately, alternative practitioners often take advantage of patients with CFS and charge them a lot of money for treatments of questionable value.

Here are my general recommendations for people with CFS:

- Take astragalus root for its antiviral and immunity-enhancing properties. I've used Astra-8, a mixture of astragalus and seven other Chinese herbs. Take three tablets twice a day. You should have no problem staying on it indefinitely.
- Take maitake mushrooms, generally available in health food stores. These are nontoxic and may speed recovery. Follow dosage on the product container.
- Take my antioxidant formula (see page 1). In addition, take 60–100 milligrams of coenzyme Q, plus a B-100 B-complex supplement.
- Eat a low-protein, low-fat, high-carbohydrate diet.
- Eat one to two cloves of raw garlic a day. Garlic is a potent antibiotic, with antibacterial and antiviral effects as well. (By the way, a clove of garlic is one of the segments making up the head or bulb. Don't eat the whole bulb!) Chop it fine and mix with food, or swallow chunks like pills.
- Be careful about joining support groups. Find a group that encourages recovery, not the idea that you will be sick forever.

Again, tell your wife not to despair. Many of my patients have recovered. I'd like to hear back from you in two to three months, after you've tried these methods.

Fighting a Cold?

Q:

I've spent too much money on all these fancy over-the-counter products for colds. Sometimes they mask the symptoms, but they don't really seem to make me better. Any other recommendations?

A:

You're absolutely right. Most of the over-the-counter products don't help you heal, even if they do stop the sniffles and headaches for a short while. I learned recently that more over-the-counter products are sold for the common cold than for any other disease. Not really surprising. Over the years, I have been collecting home remedies for colds—using myself and my family as guinea pigs. Here's what I've found works best:

Take vitamin C to prevent colds—2,000 milligrams, three times a day. You should start this now.

As soon as you start feeling cold symptoms, eat two cloves (not heads) of raw garlic. Trust me on this. You may not be kissing anyone soon, but garlic has powerful antibiotic effects. Chop it up and mix it with food, or swallow larger pieces like pills.

You can also take echinacea (*Echinacea purpurea* and related species) at the first sign of a cold or flu—like a scratchy throat or achy back. Take a dropperful of the tincture in a little warm water (or tea) four times a day. Use half doses for children.

Try sucking on zinc gluconate or zinc acetate lozenges,

which, according to a recent study, may cut the duration of a cold in half.

Finally, drink this powerful gingerroot tea for head and chest congestion, malaise, and the chills. Here's my recipe:

> Grate a 1-inch piece of peeled gingerroot. Put it in a pot with 2 cups of cold water, bring to a boil, lower heat, and simmer five minutes. Add $1/2$ teaspoon cayenne pepper (or more or less to taste) and simmer one minute more. Remove from heat. Add 2 tablespoons of fresh lemon juice, honey to taste, and 1 or 2 cloves of mashed garlic. Let cool slightly, and strain if you desire.

Then get under the covers and drink as much of it as you like. Hope you feel better.

Charmed by Colloidal Minerals?

Q:
How do you feel about taking colloidal mineral supplements?

A:
To me these supplements exemplify obnoxious, multi-level marketing in the name of natural medicine. I've received countless copies of an audiotape that advertises colloidal minerals and makes all sorts of claims. The veterinarian who pitches the stuff is said to have been nominated for the Nobel Prize in medicine. Well, anyone can write a letter to the Nobel Prize committee. I could nominate you for the Nobel Prize in medicine. I have not seen convincing evidence of therapeutic benefit from taking colloidal minerals. And these products may deliver some substances you definitely don't need—aluminum, for example. Well, I feel better after venting.

"Colloidal" means the mineral particles are of a certain size, facilitating use by the body. The marketers will tell you that their products make you live twice as long, protect you from cancer, and cure just about anything. They'll tell you that mineral deficiencies lead to a weakened immune system and cancer. You can buy the products as liquid supplements, aerosols, injectables, and vaginal douches. The literature in health food stores says they're powerful antimicrobials and immune-system stimulants; they're supposed to help cure as many as 650 different diseases. None of these claims are proven.

Some colloidal minerals have a long history as medicinals. In the nineteenth century, for example, colloidal silver was promoted as a treatment for everything from colds to rheumatism. Silver products are useful as germicidals, but over time they've been replaced by safer and more effective ones.

There is some potential for harm, as well. The body doesn't need silver, and the mineral can accumulate in tissues, causing an irreversible bluish discoloration of the skin. There are even some reports of neurological problems in people who have used oral silver products long-term.

Bottom line: I don't recommend colloidal minerals; there's no reason to think they're as good for you as they are for their marketers. Besides, you should be getting your minerals in highly usable forms from fruits and vegetables in your diet. Please eat more fruits and vegetables—organically grown, when possible.

Is Decaf Really Any Better?

Q:
How much safer is decaf than regular coffee?

A:
Although new caffeine-extraction methods seem to preserve the flavor of a good cup of coffee, decaffeinated coffee is not the safe, easy solution for java junkies. Decaf retains enough caffeine to affect sensitive people. It also contains other substances naturally found in the coffee bean that can have irritating effects on the body. For example, decaffeinated coffee can be just as tough on the stomach as regular coffee.

If you have reason to avoid coffee, you would do well to avoid decaf also. If you have any of the following conditions, stay away from both drinks: migraine, tremor, anxiety, heart palpitations, insomnia, coronary heart disease or a strong family history of it, high cholesterol, any gastrointestinal disorder, any urinary disorder, prostate trouble, fibrocystic breasts, premenstrual syndrome, tension headaches, or seizure disorder.

A study done at the University of California at Berkeley found a relationship between drinking decaf and a slightly increased risk of high cholesterol and heart disease. In that survey of about 45,500 men, regular coffee did not have the same effect.

But if you really want to have a cup of decaf, I'd recommend using only the water-extracted versions. There is concern that some traces of solvents remain in coffee decaffeinated by other methods, although the manufacturers deny it.

There are many coffee substitutes available in supermarkets and health food stores. They are made from roasted grains, roots, acorns, and other benign ingredients. I recommend Cafix, Roma, Dacopa, and Teccino. Experiment with them, or use a caffeine-free herbal tea.

Fight Depression Without Drugs?

Q:

What alternatives are there to conventional anti-depressant medications or EST (electroshock therapy)? I have tried every medical therapy possible—except EST—but still face recurrent spontaneous episodes of major depression. Are there any alternative treatments that might halt this escalating cycle?

A:

There are only two alternative treatments for depression that I have any confidence in. The first is regular aerobic exercise, which can definitely provide a long-term solution. You'll have to do at least thirty minutes of some vigorous aerobic activity at least five times a week, and be prepared to wait several weeks before you see any benefit. Aerobic exercise is a preventive as well as a treatment.

The second is an herbal treatment, called Saint-John's-wort (*Hypericum perforatum*). Saint-John's-wort is much used in Germany for the treatment of mild to moderate depression, as well as associated disturbed sleep cycles. Take 300 milligrams, three times a day, of a standardized extract containing at least 0.125 percent hypericin. Again, be prepared to wait several months before you see the full benefit.

Changes in your diet may also make a difference. Try eating less protein and fat, and more starches, fruits, and vegetables. Experiment with the following amino acid and vitamin formula, for which you can find all the ingredients in a health food store. First thing in the morning, take 1,500 milligrams of DL-phenylalanine (DLPA, an amino acid), 100 milligrams of vitamin B-6, and 500 milligrams of vitamin C, along with a piece of fruit or a small glass of juice. Don't eat again for at least an hour. (DLPA can worsen high blood pressure, so use the formula cautiously if you have this condition, and start with a dose of 100 milligrams while monitoring your blood pressure.) Take another 100 milligrams of B-6 and more vitamin C in the evening.

You say you've taken a variety of drugs for depression. In general, I think that the new generation of antidepressants, including Prozac, Zoloft, and Paxil, are less toxic and more effective than medications of the past. Collectively known as SSRIs, or selective serotonin-reuptake inhibitors, they interact with the regulating mechanism for the neurotransmitter serotonin in your brain. It's best to be cautious with any of these drugs, particularly because their makers would have you believe that no one can live a normal life without them.

Make sure you aren't taking any other medications that may contribute to depression. These include antihistamines, tranquilizers, sleeping pills, and narcotics. Recreational drugs, alcohol, and coffee can also make depression worse.

You make reference to EST—electroshock or electroconvulsive therapy. That is a last resort for the treatment of severe depression. It does work, but I hope things won't get to the point where that's your only option.

Psychiatrists tend to look at all mental problems as stemming from disordered brain chemistry; hence their emphasis on drugs. I believe that disordered moods could just as easily lead to biochemical changes in the brain, so I look elsewhere for treatments. Buddhist psychology views depression as the necessary consequence of seeking stimulation. It counsels us to cultivate emotional balance in life, rather than always seeking highs and then regretting the lows that follow. The prescription is daily meditation, and I agree this may be the best way to get at the root of depression and change it.

Does DHEA Improve Memory?

Q:
My father-in-law takes DHEA along with a few other drugs, all under a doctor's care. He was having trouble remembering things and even being able to carry on a conversation. He says DHEA helps a lot, although he doesn't think it is enhancing his memory. What does DHEA do, exactly?

A:
DHEA is a natural hormone produced by the adrenal glands, in the family of male sex hormones. Currently there is great medical interest in DHEA (dehydro-epiandrosterone), as well as a push from the supplement industry to promote it as an antiaging, antiobesity, anti-cancer remedy. Smart-drug enthusiasts think it can also protect brain cells from the degenerative changes of old age. A lot of claims, but not a lot of conclusive science as yet.

What we do know is that DHEA has a significant ana-bolic effect, which results in stronger bones and muscles and decreased body fat. It may protect health in a variety of ways. I've seen good results with DHEA in patients with autoimmune diseases like lupus. I also think it might help people with other diseases, such as asthma and rheumatoid arthritis, who have become dependent on prednisone, since it may allow them to wean their bodies off that more dan-gerous hormone. DHEA is sold as a prescription drug and by several mail-order pharmacies. Health food stores sell DHEA precursors, but they may be worthless. The extracts from wild yams will have no effect, either.

People who tout DHEA point out that we produce most of this hormone in our twenties, with production tapering off in our later years until we produce only about one-fifth as much. They suggest that supplemental DHEA beginning at age forty or fifty could improve quality of life. But evidence for DHEA's benefits is inconclusive. There was one small, six-month study at the University of California–San Diego that reported improved energy and feelings of well-being.

I'm cautious about using any hormones on a regular basis without good reason and without medical supervision. We don't know what the downside of taking supplemental DHEA may be over time. Ray Sahelian, M.D., author of *DHEA: A Practical Guide*, warns against taking high doses cavalierly and suggests consulting with a physician before trying DHEA, because it is a steroid that the body converts into potent estrogens and androgens. Side effects can include acne, facial hair growth in women, deepening of the voice, and mood changes. DHEA probably increases risk of prostate cancer and may increase risk of coronary heart disease.

If your father-in-law's chief concern is his memory, I would suggest an herbal preparation made from the leaves of the ginkgo tree (*Ginkgo biloba*). Researchers have recently begun to study the ability of ginkgo extracts to increase blood flow to the brain. You can buy this nontoxic product in any health food store. Your father-in-law could try taking two tablets or capsules three times a day with meals for memory enhancement. He might not notice any beneficial effects until he has used ginkgo for six to eight weeks.

Does Echinacea
Fight Colds?

Q:
Is echinacea helpful in the treatment of colds and flu? Does it really work as an immune system "booster" to help protect against them? What is the proper dosage? Is it the same for treatment as for prevention? What parts of the plant should be used?

A:
Echinacea (*Echinacea purpurea* and related species) is a common plant in North America, cultivated ornamentally in gardens as purple coneflower. Besides being pretty, it really does work as an immune system booster. Echinacea is very popular as a medicinal, and there are hundreds of products made from it.

There is a great deal of research from Germany showing that echinacea increases the number and activity of key white blood cells involved in immunity. It is known to boost the activity of T cells and natural killer cells and the production of interferon. The herb is versatile and very safe. Take it at the first sign of a cold or flu—symptoms like a scratchy throat or achy back.

The root contains the highest concentration of echinacea's active material, although the leaves are also potent. Some products are made from the whole plant; I prefer tinctures made from the root. At the first sign of a cold or flu, take a dropperful of the tincture in a little warm water (or tea) four times a day. Use half that much for children. Make sure the echinacea is potent by putting a bit on your tongue; if it produces a marked numbing sensation after a few minutes, it's good.

I generally don't use echinacea as a preventive, though some people do. The only time I might is if I go on a long plane flight, when the air is recirculated and unhealthy. Then I take echinacea for a couple of days beforehand. To build immunity, you may want to try echinacea at half the adult dosage and stay on it two weeks at a time.

There's a popular belief among herbalists that echinacea loses its effectiveness if it's taken continually for more than two or three weeks. But there is no evidence to support that belief, so I think you can go on taking it for as long as you think you need it.

Desperately Seeking Relief from Fleas?

Q:
I'm desperately seeking relief from flea bites and the allergic reaction I get. I have tried numerous internal and external repellents (vitamin B-12, eucalyptus, pennyroyal) to no avail. The fleas find me, bite, and cause severe itching over my entire body. This is extremely uncomfortable and upsetting as they are leaving chicken pox–like scarring that lasts for months. Have you any experience with this?

A:
This is a tough one. Fleas love the humid conditions of Hawaii, coastal California, the Gulf Coast, and the Atlantic seaboard south of Maryland. Breeding conditions there are perfect year-round, and with one hundred fleas able to produce a half-million offspring in one month, you can see why they continue to find you.

I'm sorry to say your best hope may be to fumigate your house with chemical "bombs" available at pet food stores and veterinarians' offices. (Make sure you stay out of your house during the bombing process.) In my experience, the natural repellents that you mention don't work nearly as well as chemical pesticides for severe infestations.

Pyrethrins, active insecticidal agents found in chrysanthemum extracts, will kill the fleas and degrade rapidly in the environment. They are nontoxic to humans. You will need to use these or other treatments more than once in order to kill more than one generation of fleas. Growth regulators like fenoxycarb mimic flea hormones and prevent the young larvae from becoming adult fleas.

One natural product that you might try is called Neem. It's a powerful and relatively safe insecticide obtained from a tree in India. You should be able to find it at garden stores. Also, some people dust carpets, furniture, and the crevices where fleas hide out with diatomaceous earth, which contains the fossilized "skeletons" of sea algae. Organic farmers often use it to kill insects; its sharp crystals puncture their bodies.

There are biological insecticides that you can try outdoors. Several brands available at lawn and garden stores employ nematodes—tiny worms—that feed on the flea larvae.

You don't say whether you have pets. If you do, try keeping them outside the house. Wash their bedding in hot water and detergent and keep doing so once a week. Also, there's a relatively new product available from vets called Program, which you adminster to your pet once a month. Many people have seen dramatic improvement in bad flea situations after starting to use Program.

Once you get things under control, vacuuming every other day may help remove the eggs that fleas lay in the carpet. Get rid of the vacuum bag each time, because the fleas will hatch inside. When you wash the floor, pay special attention to baseboards and areas under the furniture. Shampoo your carpets or bring in a professional steam cleaner at least twice a year. The best way to fight fleas is to keep your environment scrupulously clean.

Getting Enough
Folic Acid?

Q:

How important is folic acid? Can't I get this and other B vitamins in a balanced diet?

A:

Folic acid, the synthetic form of the B vitamin folate, is incredibly important. For one thing, folate is a key regulator of an amino acid called homocystine, a breakdown product of animal protein. A number of studies have connected high levels of homocystine in the blood to arterial disease and heart attacks. Folate helps the body eliminate homocystine from the blood. Recently, Dr. Howard Morrison, an epidemiologist in Ottawa, was able to make a direct connection between folate and heart disease. He looked at folate levels in the blood of 5,056 men who had participated in a nutrition study in the 1970s, and he found that those with low levels of the vitamin were 69 percent more likely to have died from heart problems in the years since.

Folate also has been found to prevent neural tube defects (such as spina bifida and anencephaly) in babies, caused when this structure fails to form properly. The neural tube is the embryonic tissue that later becomes the brain and spinal cord. Apparently folic acid is essential to its proper development. The Food and Drug Administration has ordered pasta, rice, and flour makers to add folic acid to their foods by January 1998 as protection against birth defects. This is partly because folic acid plays its important role in neural tube development during the first twenty-eight days of conception—usually before the woman knows she is pregnant—so it doesn't help to tell women to take vitamin supplements during pregnancy.

Folate also may be involved in preventing a whole range of chronic diseases. As the folic acid fortification rule moves into place, we may see a number of health benefits. In fact, since the Morrison study, some doctors are saying the government should double its folic acid RDA (recommended daily allowance), from 200 micrograms to 400 micrograms, to help people protect their hearts.

Folic acid is abundant in dark-green leafy vegetables, carrots, torula yeast, orange juice, asparagus, beans, and wheat germ. But as many as 90 percent of Americans don't get that protective 400 micrograms in their diet—for example, you'd have to eat two cups of steamed spinach, a cup of boiled lentils, or eight oranges every day. So it's important to take a supplement.

A few cautions, though: Some people are allergic to the folic acid in pills. Also, anyone with a history of convulsive disorders or hormone-related cancer should not take doses above 400 micrograms a day for extended periods. Finally, high levels of folate can mask the signs of vitamin B-12 deficiency. Older people and vegetarians, who are most at risk for deficiencies in B-12, should make sure they're also getting enough of that vitamin if they begin taking folic acid supplements.

Help for Halitosis?

Q:
I'm concerned about the causes and natural remedies for bad breath.

A:
The usual cause of bad breath is bacteria growing on the tongue, and sometimes around the gum line, too. There are a couple of simple ways to take care of the problem. First, try a tongue scraper. This is a metal instrument that you use to scrape your tongue once or twice a day, cleaning off bacteria. Second, you can brush your tongue with a germicidal toothpaste when you're brushing your teeth. Just take an extra thirty seconds to brush your tongue after you're done with your teeth. One such product that works well is chlorine dioxide, which is in some regular toothpastes (for instance, Oxyfresh). Or, use a toothpaste containing tea tree oil. This nontoxic oil is extracted from the leaves of *Melaleuca alternifolia*, and is a powerful disinfectant that smells a bit like eucalyptus. You can find toothpastes with tea tree oil at your local health food or herb store.

For temporary breath problems—say, when you return to work after a garlic-and-onion-laden lunch—try chewing on a bit of parsley or some fennel seeds. These will freshen your breath and also offer a nice finish to a meal. Try to stay away from products like Certs and Breath-Savers; they contain aspartame.

Bad breath can also sometimes be related to gum disease. Check your gums for signs of irritation or swelling. If you notice a problem, talk to your dentist about it (he or she may refer you to a periodontist). Constant bad breath also may be a sign of systemic illness, especially liver disease or kidney disease. If it's a systemic problem, the breath is likely to have a distinct smell. Liver problems produce a mousy odor; severe bronchial infections will smell rotten. Sinusitis and inflammation inside the nose can also cause bad breath.

I wouldn't pay much attention to the claims made about mouthwashes like Scope or Listerine. These germicidal formulas may help, but they often don't penetrate into the crevices of the tongue. That's why I prefer brushing the tongue directly.

Cure for Hangovers?

Q:
I hate getting out of bed to find myself with a splitting reminder of the night before. Is there anything that can help cure the common hangover?

A:
Alcohol is a strong toxin to both the liver and the nervous system, and it irritates the upper digestive tract and urinary system as well. The morning after a binge, you also feel the effects of dehydration. It certainly seems that everyone has a cure for a hangover: sailors claim salt water is the antidote; the Egyptians ate boiled cabbage as a preventive; today, many folks claim it's the "hair of the dog" that'll stop the hammering. Believe what you will.

I probably don't need to say that moderation is the best way to avoid hangovers. It makes sense to imbibe as much water as possible while you're drinking alcohol, to avoid dehydration. Taking aspirin before drinking, though popular, doesn't help. The best and only surefire remedy is time: as your body metabolizes the toxic overdose, symptoms subside. If you have access to pure oxygen in a canister you can try inhaling some to see if it speeds recovery, but I doubt this is practical for most people. I recommend taking a B-complex vitamin supplement plus extra thiamine (100 milligrams) to counter the B-vitamin depletion caused by alcohol. But I really don't know of any hangover treatment that works as well as putting time between yourself and the night before.

Be aware that you should pick your poison wisely. Since alcohol is exempt from most labeling requirements, it may contain additives that can trigger asthma, migraines, and other reactions. Whenever possible, choose quality brands. The extra money you pour out for a premium cocktail may tax your wallet, but will help your liver love you.

Some distilled beverages are rich in substances called congeners, toxic impurities that can greatly add to your woes. Bourbon, rum, and cognac are particularly "dirty." Champagne and some sweet wines are also notorious causers of hangovers. Vodka, being just pure alcohol and water, is the cleanest.

It's always a good idea to pace yourself, and to eat if you have more than a drink or two.

My drink of choice is sake, which seems pretty clean to me. I don't get a hangover from it, even when I drink more than normal. *Kanpai!*

Healing Remedies for Herpes?

Q:

What do you recommend for treating genital herpes? I've tried acyclovir, and I've found it interrupts the virus's behavior but does nothing for healing the body. I've also been taking L-lysine three times a day and have found this to be effective. While I'm at it: Any thoughts about treating herpes on the lips?

A:

As you learned, acyclovir is less than ideal. It's expensive, may have side effects, and merely suppresses the symptoms without correcting them. L-lysine, an amino acid present in various foods, is worth trying because it inhibits replication of the herpes virus. I recommend 500 to 1,000 milligrams a day on an empty stomach. You can enhance L-lysine's effectiveness by minimizing foods like nuts, seeds, peas, and chocolate. In my experience, I usually find L-lysine more effective with oral herpes than genital.

You might want to experiment with another natural product: red marine algae (of the family *Dumontiaceae*), marketed under the name Intracept Pro (made by In Life Energy Systems). In lab tests, red marine algae appears to inhibit the herpes virus, although definitive human tests are lacking.

Many people have seen their herpes go into complete remission as a result of changes in lifestyle and mental attitude. Others have experienced significantly fewer flare-ups after trying visualizations and mental affirmations that tell the virus it's welcome in the body as long as it stays in the dormant stage. There's definitely the possibility of living in balance with the organism even if you can't get rid of it. Let me know how red marine algae works for you.

Home Tests for HIV?

Q:
Are over-the-counter HIV tests accurate or reliable?

A:
The Food and Drug Administration approved home HIV tests after a great deal of debate. When the first tests were submitted for regulatory scrutiny, there was much concern about accuracy. On top of that, the FDA and some AIDS activists worried that people would not get the psychological help they needed when they learned the results of positive tests. This information can be extremely upsetting. People who are tested at clinics or by their doctors always receive their results in person—from a trained professional. Counseling is critical to understanding what the results mean, learning how to cope with them, and finding out about treatment (if one is infected). Many people feel there is just no substitute for face-to-face counseling.

The FDA ultimately decided that the tests were highly accurate and that they assured patient anonymity and provided appropriate counseling. It was thought that this option would allow more people to be tested and to know their HIV status, which in turn could stem the tide of new infections. In one survey, many people said they preferred the home test to going to a clinic. Men of color in particular said they were more likely to use a home test kit. And according to the Centers for Disease Control and

Prevention, 85 percent of people tested in clinics don't get counseling with the results.

If it's more convenient and you decide you don't want to talk to someone in person, I think a home test is fine. Just make sure you do make use of the counseling available by phone.

The Confide HIV testing service, from a subsidiary of Johnson & Johnson, put out the first home kit on the market. In data submitted to regulators, the kit was 99.95 percent accurate in identifying 3,940 samples of uninfected blood. It also correctly picked out all of the 150 samples infected with HIV, the virus that causes AIDS. In mid-1997, Johnson & Johnson pulled the Confide test from the market, claiming that only 90,000 tests had been processed during the previous year and that demand wasn't expected to grow. The FDA had also sent two warning letters to the company regarding the test, so it's not entirely clear why the product was pulled.

The standard Home Access test costs $29.95 for results by phone within seven days. The "express" Home Access test is $49.95 for results within three days. Call (800) HIV TEST (448-8378) for more information.

Here's how the test works: You start by reading the instructions and pretest counseling booklet, which are in both Spanish and English. Then you prick your finger with a fingerstick in the kit and collect a blood sample. You drip three drops of blood onto a test card marked with a special identification number, and you mail it to a laboratory for HIV-antibody testing. Seven days later, you call a toll-free number, day or night, for the results. If the results are negative, an automated voice tells you so. If they are positive, you talk to a live person about them, what they mean, and how to get medical care.

It's very important to stay on the phone and talk to the counselor once you get the result. Realize that false positives do occur, so if you test positive, you should get tested again. The lab will do a second test by the same method, and if that one's positive, will perform a more sophisticated test called the Western blot.

If you test positive, the counselor will tell you about a number of drugs that lengthen life expectancy. You can also find out about medical, psychological, and legal services available to you.

Also, keep in mind that a negative result doesn't mean you never have to worry about HIV again. If you're sexually active in a nonmonogamous situation, or if you inject drugs, it's important to get tested regularly. There is a "window" period of up to six months where you may be infected without the virus's showing up on a test.

And always use a condom or a dental dam to protect yourself during sexual intercourse. If you do inject drugs, use a clean needle.

How to Get Unleaded?

Q:
My son has lead poisoning. What will the treatment be?

A:
Lead poisoning in fetuses and young children is a serious problem in the United States. Even low-level lead exposure can cause hyperactivity, learning disabilities, and growth problems over time. High-level poisoning can reduce intelligence, cause severe retardation, and even lead to death. It's very important to test for lead in young children because they are so susceptible to its effects, particularly as their brains develop. Plus, there is so much lead in the environment that it is easy for them to get exposed. If your drinking water contains more than 10 parts per billion of lead, you and your family will consume enough of this heavy metal to do harm.

The most common sources of lead are water from lead pipes, flakes of lead paint inside houses and in the dirt around homes, lead glazes on pottery, and lead from older processing equipment and fuels that ends up in canned vegetables. Get rid of all known sources of lead. You should find out what your pipes are made of and get your water tested for lead content. Or you can purchase a home purifying system that will remove lead and other heavy metals. The Centers for Disease Control and Prevention suggests that every child under age six be tested for lead poisoning.

I recommend two precautions to reduce the chance of

ingesting lead from household water. First, let the water
run from the tap for three to five minutes after any period
of nonuse. Second, don't draw water from the hot tap—
even for cooking—because hot water leaches out impurities much more readily than cold, and because it is likely
to have sat for long periods in the hot-water tank. In fact,
no matter what your pipes are made of, water from the
hot tap is unfit for human consumption.

If you detect lead poisoning early, there are ways to
counter it. The American Association of Naturopathic
Physicians recommends a nutritional approach. The antioxidants—vitamins A, C, and E, plus selenium—can
help detoxify the body and protect nerve tissue from
damage. Zinc and vitamin C help reduce harm from the
lead, and vitamin A may counter infections that lead-
poisoned children tend to suffer. The association also
suggests a regimen of herbs and amino acids to detoxify
the liver.

If lead poisoning is confirmed, I would be inclined to
go for the conventional treatment: chelation therapy.
Injected or oral chelating agents bond with lead, allowing
the child to excrete the metal in his or her urine. The
newest oral medicine is Succimer, or DMSA. The treatment normally lasts nineteen days and should go no
longer than three weeks. Side effects of chelation therapy
can include rash, nausea, and a loss of appetite, but the
benefits of getting the lead out are much greater than the
risks of therapy.

How to Lick
Lyme Disease?

Q:
We live in a wooded area in central Wisconsin and often have deer in our backyard. What is a safe way to protect our two-year-old son and ourselves from ticks? Are products like Deep Woods Off! safe for small children? Our son already has had two ticks on him this year. (I don't think they were deer ticks as they were pretty large.) Any info on ticks and Lyme disease would be appreciated.

A:
Lyme disease is an infection caused by an organism called *Borrelia burgdorferi*. It's named after Old Lyme, Connecticut, where doctors discovered the disease when they thought they had an epidemic of juvenile rheumatoid arthritis. There were about 8,000 cases of it in the United States in 1993, the most recent year for which I have figures.

Lyme disease presents a curious situation. There's a tremendous fascination with it as an exotic illness. And people are fearful of it because the symptoms can persist years after infection, even with treatment. So there's a tendency to rush to this diagnosis whenever patients have strange, persistent symptoms.

At the same time, a definitive diagnosis is often missed. Some physicians don't think to look for it and thus fail to give the proper treatment. To further complicate matters, we don't have a conclusive test for Lyme

47

disease and there's no way of being sure it is the cause of any specific symptom.

Lyme disease is usually treated with up to one month of antibiotics. If these are administered at the right time and in the right way, they should eradicate the organism.

If the disease is left untreated, about two-thirds of people infected develop recurring bouts of arthritis, sometimes years after the initial infection. The disease also has been associated with neurological symptoms, although it's not clear how severe they may be.

As you say, deer ticks host the organism. Deer, deer mice, and field mice carry the ticks, which are so small, they're practically invisible until fully engorged with blood—and then they are still hard to see. So the ticks you saw were not deer ticks. You should find out whether deer ticks are present in your area, and if so, whether they carry the bacteria that causes Lyme disease.

Generally, I don't recommend any chemical pesticides. The only safe insecticide is pyrethrum, which is made from the heads of certain chrysanthemums. In areas where the disease is really prevalent, like Long Island and Connecticut, the best prevention is to wear protective clothing when you go out into the woods. Wear light colors and long sleeves, and tuck your pants into your socks. When you get back, wash immediately and keep an eye out for anything unusual on your body.

If you do have any odd symptoms like strange skin rashes, fever, or joint pain, go to a doctor who is knowledgeable about diagnosing and treating Lyme disease. The typical presentation is a rash in concentric rings, like a bull's-eye. But in many cases it is not present.

When to Get a Mammogram?

Q:
I'm totally confused by recent medical reports providing conflicting information about when women should go for mammograms. In your opinion, at what age should women start getting them on a regular basis?

A:
I don't blame you for your confusion. Public health authorities are at odds over this question, and the debate isn't over yet. Meanwhile, women are left in the dark on how best to take care of themselves.

The issue in question is whether women in their forties should get routine mammograms to screen for breast cancer in its earliest stages. Very recently, the American Cancer Society issued new guidelines for mammograms, recommending that women in their forties have the cancer screening performed annually. Previous guidelines recommended mammograms every one to two years starting at age forty, and every year beginning at age fifty. The panel said that annual mammograms for women in their forties could save as many as 10,000 lives in the next five years.

According to Dr. Marilyn Leitch, an oncologist at the University of Texas Southwestern Medical Center, "The current average two-year interval between mammograms may be too long in this age group and their faster-growing cancers."

49

Just when a woman should begin mammography screening has been hotly debated since 1993, when the National Cancer Institute (of the National Institutes of Health) backed off its guideline that women should begin the screenings at age forty. In 1996 the issue took on new significance with the appearance of mixed data about the benefits of screening women in their forties.

In my opinion, one of the most important things to keep in mind is that the effectiveness of a mammogram as a diagnostic technique depends entirely on the experience and skill of the person who reads it. Be sure to go to an expert. If you don't know whom to call, contact the American Cancer Society at (800) ACS-2345 (227-2345). It's also my experience that mammograms do pick up tiny cancers that if left until palpable would be much more serious and life-threatening. I know several women whose lives were saved by early detection of breast cancer after a mammogram.

The downside, of course, is the amount of radiation involved. As readers know, I am opposed to needless exposure to X-ray radiation. The ultimate conclusion of the NIH panel is that every woman needs to decide for herself whether to get a mammogram and at what age; this decision should be based on her family history and risk profile.

Latest on Melatonin?

Q:
What do you think of melatonin? Is 3 milligrams a normal dose?

A:
Melatonin is the first and only effective remedy for jet lag, and I recommend it for that purpose (it's even effective for west-to-east travel, which many people find harder). It's also useful as an occasional remedy for insomnia—especially for people working shifts—or for disturbed sleep cycles. If you go through periods where you're dead tired at 7 P.M. and then awake at, say, 11 P.M., melatonin might change your cycle, allowing you to go to sleep at a better time and sleep for the whole night. For these uses, taking melatonin for only one or two nights might be sufficient.

But evidence for melatonin's effects as an immune-booster and a chemical fountain of youth is lacking—popular books and articles notwithstanding. Because it is a brain hormone, secreted by the pineal gland, with very general effects on the body, I'm wary about recommending it for use on a regular basis over long periods of time.

You should be aware that the quality of melatonin products on the market is uneven, and many dosage forms are too high. A 1 milligram tablet taken sublingually (under the tongue) is probably more than enough for any use. The best book on the topic is *Melatonin*, by Russel J. Reiter, Ph.D., and Jo Robinson.

Help for Migraines?

Q:
What is the best natural cure for migraine headaches?

A:
Migraines are very unpleasant, often putting people out of action for days at a time as well as frustrating doctors, who frequently find that their arsenal of medications doesn't do the job. Western doctors prescribe to migraine sufferers many strong drugs that can do more harm than good. Allergy, hormonal fluctuations, stress, and heredity are all factors that trigger attacks. My recommendations include:

- Eliminate coffee and decaf (and other sources of caffeine). Once a patient is off caffeine, coffee can be used as a treatment. Drink one or two cups of strong coffee at the first sign of an attack, then go lie down in a dark room.
- Eliminate other dietary triggers like chocolate, red wine (sometimes white wine, too), strong-flavored cheeses, fermented foods (like soy sauce and miso), sardines, anchovies, and pickled herring.
- As a preventive, take feverfew (*Tanacetum parthenium*) herb, which is a little plant related to chrysanthemum. You can buy a plant at a local nursery—it's a common ornamental—and chew a few leaves a day (be warned: they don't taste great), or you can buy a standardized extract at any health food store. Read the label to make

sure it has the necessary active components, parthenolides, in it. One or two tablets or capsules a day will significantly reduce the frequency of migraines in many people. You can stay on feverfew indefinitely.

- Take a course of biofeedback training and learn how to raise the temperature of your hands. This will be a helpful tool to abort a headache at the start of an attack. To find a practitioner near you, look in the yellow pages or contact the Biofeedback Certification Institute of America.
- Use prescription medications sparingly. Try ergotamine to abort migraine attacks; it is a powerful constrictor of arteries that in order to work must be used at the first sign of an attack.
- Don't take Fiorinal on a regular basis. Many doctors prescribe it like candy to migraine sufferers without telling them that it contains an addictive downer (butalbital) and caffeine, as well as aspirin. Don't take prednisone or steroids to prevent attacks; the potential dangers outweigh the benefits.

If you continue to have attacks, think about changing the way you think about your headaches. Migraines are like an electrical storm in the brain—violent and disruptive—but leading to a calm, clear state in the end. It's not so bad to have a headache once in a while; it actually can be a good excuse to drop routines, focus inwardly, and let stress dissipate. If you can come to accept the migraines in this way, they may occur less frequently.

How Good
Are Multis?

Q:
I'd like your opinion on multivitamins. I'm in good health but can't often eat right. Is a good multivitamin advisable? And if so, what should I look for? Is there any difference between different brands of the exact same vitamins? What's the best way to compare them?

A:
If you're not eating regularly, if your diet is not rich in fresh foods, and if you don't get plenty of fruits and vegetables, a multivitamin is an easy solution. It's better to take your vitamin cocktail in stages throughout the day, but I'm not opposed to taking your daily requirement all at once in one capsule, pill, or tablet after your biggest meal.

Some precautions: I would check the doses to make sure you're getting enough antioxidants. That would be 25,000 IU beta-carotene (preferably with other carotenes such as alpha-carotene, lutein, zeaxanthin, and lycopene), 400 IU of natural vitamin E (twice that much if you're over forty), and 2,000 milligrams of vitamin C, plus 200 micrograms of selenium a day. If not, take extra supplements to make up the difference.

It's also possible to get too much of some things in a multivitamin. You don't want more than 400 micrograms a day of folic acid, because then you risk masking a vitamin B-12 deficiency without added benefits from the folic acid. And make sure there's no iron in there, if you're not a woman of menstruating age or a person with proven iron-

54

deficiency anemia. Iron is an oxidizing agent that can promote cancer and heart disease, and the body has no way of eliminating excess amounts except through blood loss.

I don't think those vitamin packs are worth it. You can make up your own packs, if you want. Or if it's the convenience you're after, a multivitamin probably makes more sense.

In general, when shopping for the vitamins, there really aren't any buzzwords to look for. Just use the same common sense you might use when looking for a bottle of juice for lunch, or the right flour for the bread you're baking. You want products free of dyes, preservatives, and nonessential additives. And you might as well check out the cheapest ones that are free of additives first.

Read the labels. See whether the vitamin is in the form you like—a big capsule, a soft gel capsule, or a tablet. Look at the dose, and make sure the cheapest isn't just a lower amount of the vitamin encased in the same number of tablets. And make sure you know the desired dose. For instance, you can buy a calcium supplement only to find out you need six tablets in order to get the dose you want. Once I got a B-50 B-complex home and then realized that it provided only 200 milligrams a day of folic acid—half the daily amount I recommend.

Generally, the difference between natural and synthetic vitamins is not important. An exception is vitamin E. Most of the vitamin E you see on store shelves is synthetic, noted as dl-alpha tocopherol on the label. Don't buy it. Instead, go for natural vitamin E, or d-alpha tocopherol, combined with other tocopherols. Once you find a brand you like for a particular vitamin, stick with it.

You'll find there are enormous differences in pricing. I've gotten my best deals from Trader Joe's and some of the mail-order discount houses. It's worth doing some research to find reliable, low-priced sources. Two places to try are L&H Vitamins and The Vitamin Shoppe.

What's Olestra All About?

Q:
I need info on olestra. What are the side effects? Does it take away nutrients from your system? I have heard that it flushes through the system and depletes vitamins. True?

A:
Olestra is a relatively new product that tastes and feels like fat but doesn't add fat or calories to the body because it's indigestible. Recently, the Center for Science in the Public Interest, a consumer group, asked the FDA to withdraw its recent approval of olestra because a study found that 20 percent of people who ate potato chips made with olestra had stomach problems; for 3 percent of them the problems were severe.

Olestra, manufactured by Procter & Gamble as Olean, is made with two natural products: sugar and vegetable oil. P&G replaces the glycerol in a normal fat with sucrose, then adds six, seven, or eight fatty acids instead of the three found in regular fat. What does this mean? Well, the resulting compound is too big to get into the bloodstream through the small intestine, so it really does flush through the system, as you say.

A one-ounce serving of regular potato chips contains about 150 calories and 10 grams of fat. Cooked in olestra, the same chips will contain about 70 calories and no fat.

The FDA approved olestra for use in potato chips, cheese puffs, crackers, and other salty snacks. P&G spent more than $200 million testing olestra to get it through regulatory scrutiny, but it is still under investigation for its long-term effects.

The studies found that olestra prevents absorption of vitamins A, D, E, and K, which hook onto the fat substitute and ride along as it passes through the intestine. The FDA required P&G to compensate by adding those vitamins to products containing olestra.

The fake fat also drags beta-carotene and other carotenoids along with it through the intestine and out of the body. Carotenoids may help prevent many kinds of cancer and other diseases, and some nutritionists have said they are concerned about the long-term impact of carotenoid loss due to olestra. Such questions are especially important since olestra could represent a significant change to the American diet, considering the amount of fatty snacks people eat.

Other recorded side effects from olestra include bowel-function disruptions such as cramping, gas, diarrhea, and a problem euphemistically called "anal leakage."

The most pertinent question about olestra, though, is whether its benefits outweigh its potential hazards. Sugar substitutes haven't helped anyone lose weight. Whether fat substitutes will is not clear. I would say if you're going to consume olestra, do it moderately and cautiously until there's more information about it.

How to Soothe the Poison Ivy Itch?

Q:
What is the best way to cure or alleviate the itchiness of poison ivy or oak?

A:
About half the population is susceptible to poison ivy, poison oak, and poison sumac, all members of the genus *Rhus*. The itching, blistering reaction you get from these plants is caused by a T-cell response to urushiol, the allergenic component of the oil the plants secrete. If you think you're one of the lucky ones who happen to be immune, beware: allergy to these plants can come and go quite suddenly.

The reaction usually occurs thirty-six to forty-eight hours after contact and lasts for about two weeks. You won't spread the rash by scratching the blisters, but it can spread internally around the body and surface in unexpected places.

Of course, the best defense against this family of plants is to learn how to recognize its members and avoid them. They can grow as a shrub or vine, and can be spotted by their characteristic clusters of three leaflets per leaf. These can be shiny green, red-green, or red, depending on the season. If you do touch one of the plants, wash the oil off with soap and water within twenty to thirty minutes of contact. After that, the oil soaks into the skin. Watch and wash your pets, too. One common way

to get the rash is to touch a dog that has rubbed up
against a plant and had the resin transferred to its coat.

Tecnu sells a very effective over-the-counter product
that will remove the oils of poison oak, ivy, or sumac
from the skin up to twenty-four hours after contact. The
company also makes a protective lotion that you can put
on your skin before you go out in the woods.

The absolute best treatment I know for poison ivy is to
get in the shower and run hot water—as hot as you can
stand—over the affected area for five to ten minutes. This
seems counterintuitive, because it will increase the itching. But after a few minutes, the nervous circuits seem to
get overloaded and the itching stops for a long time. If
you conscientiously repeat the hot water treatment whenever the itching returns, the whole reaction completes its
cycle rapidly and your skin will return to normal.

While hot water works better than anything, you also
can use calamine lotion as a topical treatment if you
wish. I strongly recommend against taking oral prednisone or other steroids unless there are very severe
symptoms, such as fever or difficulty in urinating. Don't
use topical steroids, either. Steroids are toxic drugs that
should be saved for serious conditions, not minor ones,
since they suppress the immune system.

Commit to Quit Smoking?

Q:
I know I should quit. I just can't seem to. I desperately need help.

A:
I know that many smokers stare at themselves in the mirror, asking, "How do I quit?" It's hard. Tobacco, in the form of cigarettes, is the most addictive drug in the world—and that says a lot. There are two reasons for this: Nicotine is one of the strongest stimulants known, and smoking is one of the most efficient drug-delivery systems. Smoking actually puts drugs into the brain more directly than intravenous injection.

In the early part of this century, cigarette smoking was accepted, and was even considered healthy and glamorous. It was seen as a way to promote mental acuity, efficiency, and relaxation. It is true that one of the "benefits" of smoking is brief relief of internal tension; unfortunately, within twenty minutes tension returns, requiring another fix.

Low-tar, low-nicotine cigarettes offer no great advantages. People tend to smoke more of them, or inhale more deeply to get the same amount of nicotine. Pipes and cigars, if the smoke is not inhaled, do not cause lung cancer and emphysema, but they do increase the risk of oral cancer (as do snuff and chewing tobacco).

I feel so strongly about people not smoking that I will not accept patients who are users unless they have made a commitment to try to quit. There are many programs available to help you do so: acupuncture, hypnotherapy, and support groups. There are also a slew of new devices—nicotine patches and gum, for instance—on the market that work for some. None of these methods works reliably for everyone. Most successful quitters do it on their own after one or more unsuccessful attempts. Going "cold turkey" also seems to work better than gradually cutting down.

Don't get discouraged. If you can't quit today, you may be able to tomorrow. You want to be motivated. You need to do this for yourself, not because someone else wants you to. Remember: You get credit for every attempt you make. In fact, the best predictor for success is making attempts to quit.

If you smoke, do this breathing exercise. It will help motivate you to quit and help you with your cravings for cigarettes. Here's how to start.

1. Sit with your back straight. Place the tip of your tongue against the ridge of tissue behind your upper front teeth, and keep it there throughout the exercise.
2. Exhale completely though your mouth, making a *whoosh* sound.
3. Close your mouth and inhale quietly through your nose to a mental count of four.
4. Hold your breath for a count of seven.
5. Exhale completely through your mouth, again making a *whoosh* sound, to a count of eight.
6. This is one breath. Now inhale again and repeat the cycle three more times.

If you smoke, you should take antioxidant vitamins and minerals (see page 1), which to some extent can reverse the changes in respiratory tissue caused by smoking, and so help protect against lung cancer. Also, increase your intake of dietary sources of carotene (carrots, sweet potatoes, yellow squash, and leafy green vegetables).

Good luck, and please set a date for your next attempt to quit.

Red Wine for a
Healthy Heart?

Q:

What are the pros and cons of drinking red wine?

A:

The wine industry has benefited tremendously from reports that moderate drinking of red wine can lower the risk of coronary heart disease. After *60 Minutes* reported on the "French Paradox" in 1991, sales of cabernet and merlot soared.

The French Paradox was first discovered when epidemiologists tried to explain the low death rates from heart disease in France in spite of a very high-fat, high-cholesterol diet. Various studies followed that showed an association between drinking red wine and a heart attack risk that was 25 to 40 percent lower. *60 Minutes* followed up with a report from the Copenhagen City Heart Study of 13,000 people over ten years: the researchers had concluded that teetotalers had twice as much risk of dying from heart disease as people who drank wine every day.

The exact mechanism isn't known, but the most popular explanation credits the red pigments in grape skins. These pigments belong to a family of compounds called proanthocyanidins, which are powerful antioxidants. If this is the primary action, however, you would get the same benefits from drinking red grape juice or eating enough red and purple fruit (certain grapes, plums, and blueberries).

The tannins in red wine also can hinder the platelet

cells in the blood from clumping together and triggering a heart attack. Plus, studies have found that any alcohol can raise levels of HDL—the protective form of cholesterol—and also inhibit platelet clumping.

But let's not forget that alcohol is toxic to the liver and to the nervous system. Most wines also contain a variety of additives, such as sulfites, which may be harmful to your health. If you're going to be a regular wine drinker, I'd recommend drinking it in moderation and selecting an organic product if possible. There is an increasing market for organic wines, produced both domestically and abroad.

I personally don't like red wine, because I think I'm allergic to something in it. It gives me a stuffy nose and a sour stomach. Red wine is a common allergen that can trigger migraine headaches as well as nasal and gastric disturbances. But again, this may have more to do with additives in wine than the wine itself, which is another reason to look for organic sources.

Seeking News on Selenium?

Q:

I've been reading about selenium in the newspaper a lot these days. Can it really prevent cancer?

A:

The recent study about selenium that came out of the University of Arizona caused quite a stir. For a long time, people have believed that selenium protects against cancer, heart ailments, and other diseases. But studies on the subject were in disagreement. So the Arizona Cancer Center at the University of Arizona in Tucson, where I teach, planned a randomized trial to study the ability of selenium supplements to protect against two skin cancers: basal cell carcinoma and squamous cell carcinoma. Dr. Larry Clark and a team of researchers recruited 1,312 patients from the eastern coastal plain of the United States, where selenium levels in the soil and crops are low, and skin cancer rates are high. All of the patients had a history of skin cancer. Half of the group received sugar pills every day for an average of 4.5 years, and the other half took 200 micrograms of selenium in supplement form each day.

Clark found that the selenium supplements didn't have any effect on skin cancers. But halfway through the study, the researchers decided to look at other types of cancers and cancer mortality in general. At the end of the study, they had some dramatic results. The people who had taken selenium had 63 percent fewer prostate cancers, 58 percent fewer colorectal cancers, and 46 percent fewer lung cancers than the rest of the group. Overall, there were 39 percent fewer new cancers among those taking selenium. And altogether, half as many died from their cancer. The selenium seemed to be so beneficial, the researchers stopped the blinded phase of the trial early.

There are several possible mechanisms for the protective effect of selenium. Selenium activates an enzyme in the body called glutathione peroxidase that protects against the formation of free radicals—those loose molecular cannons that can damage DNA. In this situation, selenium may work interchangeably (and in synergy) with vitamin E. In test-tube studies, selenium inhibited tumor growth and regulated the natural life span of cells, ensuring that they died when they were supposed to instead of turning "immortal" and hence malignant. Because of this particular action, the University of Arizona researchers say that selenium could be effective within a fairly short time frame.

There were some weaknesses in this study, among them the fact that few women were included. Because the results are not consistent with those of other studies (using lower doses), the researchers and other cancer specialists are calling for further randomized trials before any national recommendations are made about selenium supplementation.

I'm all for that. But in the meantime, I will continue to take my 200 micrograms of selenium a day—the same dose used in the study—and I suggest that you do, too. Excess selenium has been associated with toxicity, so don't go overboard. If you're not fond of popping pills, you can get 120 micrograms of selenium in just one Brazil nut. But buy the shelled kind—they're grown in a central region of Brazil where the soil is richest in selenium. Other good sources are tuna fish, seafood, wheat germ, and bran.

A Proven Sex-Drive Enhancer?

Q:
Is there anything I can take to boost my sex drive? I'm female.

A:
Of course, people have been asking this question for centuries. Curiously enough, a proven sex-drive enhancer for women is the male hormone testosterone. Women produce their own testosterone, and reputable scientific studies show that tiny additional amounts can increase libido dramatically. One testosterone product, formulated for women in menopause, is called Estratest; it also contains estrogen. If you're interested in trying it, consult a gynecologist.

An herbal possibility for women is the Mexican plant damiana (*Turnera diffusa*), which has a reputation as a female aphrodisiac. Not that much is known about it, but you can find damiana preparations in health food stores. Again, follow dosage recommendations on the label. Whichever of these appeals to you, try it for a few months and see what it can do for you. If it works, great. If not, there's no point in continuing the treatment.

But before spending money on substances like these, you might want to consider other ways to boost sexual energy. Both physical and mental well-being are important to healthy sex. Think about the interplay of emotional charge, mental imagery, and body responses associated with sex. Hypnotherapy and guided imagery therapy can help you make the most of the mind-body connection in overcoming sexual problems. Many experts, myself included, say the greatest aphrodisiac is the human mind.

Cancer-Killing Sharks?

Q:
What do you know about cancer patients using shark cartilage? How does it work to help treat the cancer?

A:
Shark cartilage has become popular as an arthritis treatment and a therapy for cancer and AIDS. I haven't seen any good scientific evidence that it works, just anecdotal reports and suggestive laboratory studies. The theory is that shark cartilage contains substances that inhibit the proliferation of new blood vessels that tumors need in order to continue to grow. Mainstream scientists have isolated several compounds from shark tissue, notably squalamine, that do have this effect. But the shark anti-tumor substances they are investigating aren't found in the cartilage. Furthermore, even if there are beneficial substances in the cartilage, I'm not convinced the commercial capsules provide them in a form the body can absorb.

Most scientists object strongly to the intense promotion and commercialization of shark cartilage, because there is so little evidence of its efficacy. Meanwhile, its popularity has helped decimate shark populations.

When considering alternative treatments for cancer, it's wise to seek good published data on outcomes from their use. If you can't find published data, ask to see statistical data from providers. Look particularly for any risk of toxicity or harm. And finally, ask to talk with patients who have undergone the alternative therapy. If you have cancer, it is important to work to improve overall health and resistance on all levels. A book on alternative cancer therapies I recommend to my cancer patients is *Choices in Healing*, by Michael Lerner.

Ouch! Relief for a Sprain?

Q:
I sprained my ankle four weeks ago. The swelling shrank considerably at first, but has remained on a plateau for the past three weeks and does not appear to be getting any better. What can I do for it? Do bad sprains normally take a long time to heal?

A:
The swelling of sprains should go down fairly quickly. If it doesn't, there may be some reason why the fluid is obstructed.

I have two suggestions. First, try acupuncture treatment. I have found acupuncture to work very effectively, especially for swollen knees; it reduces pain and speeds healing.

Second, take supplements of bromelain. This is a pineapple enzyme that's used by some sports doctors. I've seen it dramatically reduce swellings from injuries. You can buy it in capsules from health food stores. The dose is 200 to 400 milligrams, three times a day. Take it between meals, on an empty stomach—at least ninety minutes before or three hours after eating. Some people are allergic to bromelain, so stop using it if you develop any itching.

The best way to reduce swelling and blood flow during the first twenty-four hours after a sprain is to put ice on it right away. You can buy wraparound ice packs or just use a bag of frozen peas or some ice cubes in a towel. Try to keep the ice on as much as possible for the first few hours; after that, intermittent applications may be helpful. After twenty-four hours, you can start alternating heat and cold. Protect the sprain from further injury by using a wraparound bandage.

Either tincture of arnica or DMSO may ease the pain and swelling. Arnica is a plant native to the high mountains of western North America that is crushed whole and soaked in alcohol. Rub it in gently, but not into broken skin. Don't ingest tincture of arnica, it's toxic. But you can take homeopathic arnica tablets in the 30× potency. Start with four tablets as soon as possible after the injury, then four more every hour for the first day. Place the tablets under your tongue and let them dissolve. The next day, take four tablets every two hours. Then, the following day, cut back to four tablets four times a day. You may continue this for four or five days.

DMSO, or dimethyl sulfoxide, is a chemical made from wood pulp. It penetrates the skin and promotes healing. Paint a 70 percent solution of DMSO on the sore area with cotton and let it dry. You may feel warmth or stinging, and experience a garlicky taste in your mouth. Try it three times a day for three days. If there is no improvement, stop using it. If you do feel some improvement, apply DMSO twice a day for three more days, then once a day for a final three days.

Blocking Sunburn Damage?

Q:
After shaving my head I spent a weekend in the Rocky Mountain sun. Despite putting on an SPF-30 sunscreen, I woke up Monday morning with a blistering, crusty, pus-spewing top. Now it's better and the skin is just peeling, but do I have anything to be concerned about?

A:
Ouch.

The incidence of skin cancer is rising at an alarming rate, with ultraviolet (UV) radiation from the sun the major cause. One reason may be the weakening effect of atmospheric pollution on the Earth's protective ozone layer, which allows more intense solar radiation to reach us. Even though UV waves are longer and have less energy than ionizing forms of radiation like X rays, they are still powerful enough to penetrate living cells and cause DNA damage. UV radiation doesn't just hurt the skin; it can contribute to the loss of vision as you grow older by damaging the retina (macular degeneration) and the lens (cataract).

I always recommend protecting yourself in as many ways as possible. Stay out of the sun when it's at a high angle in the sky; this is when the UV rays are more energetic and more numerous (from 10 A.M. to 4 P.M.). Choose clothing that covers your skin—brimmed hats, lightweight, long-sleeve shirts. Use a powerful sunscreen (SPF-15, at least) and wear UV-protective sunglasses.

And, finally, take antioxidants to help block the chemical reactions that can trigger cancer's uncontrolled cell growth. Living in the Arizona desert, I have to follow this advice year-round.

Cancer risks increase with cumulative exposure, so you should definitely avoid getting another burn on your head. The more bad burns you get, especially in your teenage years and in your twenties, the higher your risk of skin cancer as you age. If you stop getting burned, you will lessen the danger.

Most dermatologists say it's a good idea to get in the habit of putting a high-SPF sunscreen on every morning. I agree. But as you've found, sunscreen can give you a false sense of protection. Just because you're wearing sunscreen, don't assume you can spend unlimited time in the sun. It's still good to be careful.

An old-fashioned sunscreen that is still effective is zinc oxide. This is an opaque cream that provides a mechanical barrier to sunlight. (It's now available in neon colors as well as in white.) It works extremely well, but most people don't want to walk around with their faces completely white (or electric blue).

If you do get burned, aloe is probably the most soothing treatment. You can buy bottles of the pure gel in health food stores or grow the plants around your house.

Help for Tummy Trouble?

Q:
People like me with stomach complaints such as heartburn, abdominal bloating, or gas pains are generously prescribed drugs such as Pepcid, Zantac, Tagamet, or Prilosec. Most of these drugs have potential long-term side effects, usually underplayed by Western doctors. Could you recommend gentler, natural remedies for these problems? Also, what lifestyle changes may help?

A:
Digestive disorders often can be traced to poor eating habits and stress. The gastrointestinal tract is very susceptible to the disturbing influence of stress, because it relies on complex coordination by the autonomic nervous system.

The licorice extract DGL (deglycyrrhizinated licorice) is an excellent natural remedy for all the problems you mention. DGL increases the mucous coating of the stomach, making it more resistant to the effects of acid. It is nontoxic and inexpensive, and it works better than prescription drugs. The prescription drugs act by suppressing acid production in the stomach. The problem with this approach is that you're not really getting to the root problem. As soon as you stop taking these drugs, there's going to be a rebound production of acid. If you deal with the problem by using DGL, you increase the body's defensive strength.

DGL is available as tablets or powder. Chew one to

two tablets or take $1/4$ teaspoon of the powder fifteen minutes before meals and again at bedtime. Allow the material to dissolve slowly in your mouth and run down your throat.

For stomach problems generally, a number of herbal remedies can help. Peppermint tea is wonderful for nausea, indigestion, and some cases of heartburn (but because it relaxes the sphincter where the esophagus joins the stomach, it can worsen esophageal reflux syndrome, in which stomach acid irritates the lower esophagus). In general, it soothes the lining of the digestive tract. Buy pure peppermint tea, brew it in a covered container to retain the volatile components, and drink it hot or iced. Chamomile is also excellent for heartburn and indigestion, and will not aggravate esophageal reflux. You can buy it in tea bags in the supermarket. Steep in hot water in a covered container for ten minutes, and then enjoy.

I also feel strongly that people with stomach problems should not rely solely on remedies. Try looking for the causes of your problems, which probably have to do with excess consumption of stomach irritants like coffee, other forms of caffeine, decaffeinated coffee, alcohol, and foods (or food combinations) that you don't tolerate well. Smoking is another cause of stomach distress. I'd encourage you to make some dietary experiments to see if you can reduce symptoms and thereby eliminate the problem. A simple rule: Pay attention to—and stop eating—what makes your stomach hurt. Try eating smaller amounts more frequently. And work on reducing stress in your life.

Walking for Your Life?

Q:

Is it true that walking is almost equal to jogging as an aerobic exercise?

A:

I'm a great proponent of walking. Not only is it almost equal to jogging in terms of getting your heart pumping, but I think research eventually will show that it's superior in terms of overall health benefits. There are lots of reasons to prefer walking to just about any other form of exercise. First of all, everyone knows how to do it and it doesn't require any equipment. Second, you can do it anywhere. Third, the risk of injury is far less than for any other kind of aerobic exercise.

With jogging, the risk of injury is high. A person who jogs is also more likely to become exercise-dependent or to misuse exercise. People who really go for the endorphin high are often tempted to run through the pain—and then wind up being unable to exercise at all.

I will often take a walk in the morning after I meditate. Or sometimes, in the afternoon, I walk around the ranch where I live. If I'm in a city like New York or San Francisco, I try to do as much walking as possible. Obviously, San Francisco is great because of the hills. In New York walking is also great because the people-watching is so interesting.

Walking can be meditative and relaxing. You can take in the sights or listen to something on a Walkman.

Walking exercises your brain as well as your body; it's a cross-patterned movement (right arm moves forward with the left leg) that generates harmonizing electrical activity in your brain.

I find that good running shoes with cushioned soles are best for walking. But experiment—find out what works for you. If you walk up a long, gradual hill or walk at a good clip, you can get your heart and respiratory rate high enough for aerobic benefit. Maintain good posture and be sure to swing your arms as you go. I recommend forty-five minutes a day, every day if possible. That's about three miles. Do it at least five times a week.

What's the Best Water Filter?

Q:

I know there are a lot of contaminants and toxins in water these days. What do you recommend for a water filter?

A:

Water quality varies from place to place, so you may want to have your water tested to see what impurities it contains. This could affect your choice of a filter, and help you decide whether you actually need one. The price is steep, though: It can easily cost more than $100 to test for a range of contaminants.

Chlorine and lead are the two most common contaminants in water. Chlorine produces by-products that contribute to cancer and birth defects. The chemical itself may also contribute to heart disease. As for lead, even very small amounts can cause serious harm. High-level poisoning can cause organ damage and stunt the nervous system, causing mental retardation.

In many cities now, public health officials are also finding water contaminated with *Cryptosporidium*, a microbe that can cause great harm to people with compromised immune systems. So a filtration system might be essential. Also, remember that ice cubes should be made from purified water—not water from the tap.

Be sure to check out the different kinds of filtration systems available, how often you need to change the filter, how much the replacements cost, and how difficult they are to install. Filtration systems can vary greatly in quality, efficiency, and price. The cost and trouble of keeping them maintained is an important consideration.

There are six systems available for purifying water. None of them is perfect. Each has distinct strengths and drawbacks. Always read the labeling on the product to see what exactly it claims to filter out.

Steam distillation is the surest method. Water is heated to boiling, the steam collected and cooled until it condenses again without the impurities. This method works, but it's slow, uses lots of power, and causes the water to taste flat. Distillation also will not remove some volatile organic compounds, which boil over with the steam.

Carbon filtration is probably the most popular system. Units containing specially prepared, porous carbon attach under the sink or at the tap. Carbon filtration is good for removing chlorine, toxic organic molecules, and bad tastes from water, but it doesn't capture heavy metals or minerals. The system is fast, but it stops working as soon as the carbon becomes saturated with contaminants. Also, as the carbon collects organic matter, it starts to become a breeding place for bacteria. The bacteria shoot out into your first glass of water of the day, unless you take a minute to flush water through the filter first.

Ion exchange rids water of dissolved minerals and toxic metals, but it is less efficient at removing organic molecules. It works through charged particles in the filter that exchange themselves for charged particles in the water. These filters normally employ sodium in the exchange, so unless there's another process to remove it later, you could end up with harmful levels of sodium in the purified water. This method also corrodes pipes, and can cause high levels of copper, iron, and lead in drinking water. I don't recommend it.

Purifiers that use ultraviolet light to kill microorganisms have no effect on chemical toxins.

In the past, I used a system called reverse osmosis (RO). RO removes minerals and toxic heavy metals like lead, along with the organic contaminants (including

Cryptosporidium). In an RO unit, water pressure forces water through an osmotic membrane (also called a semi-permeable membrane, because the holes allow small water molecules, but not contaminant molecules, to pass through). Bacteria are blocked out, and they don't grow on the filter. All things considered, I think this is the best way to go. However, you should know that the process is slow, and wastes a lot of water, which is why I finally stopped using it. RO water is very corrosive to pipes, so place the system near the tap.

I'm now in favor of a system that combines a solid carbon block filter with a copper-zinc alloy called KDF. This dual system removes most impurities and is affordable and simple. The KDF puts small amounts of copper and zinc into the water, which is healthful.

Natural Help for Yeast Infections?

Q:

What do I do about recurring yeast infections? I've had them for over twenty years.

A:

Many women suffer from frequent vaginal yeast infections, which can indicate an underlying metabolic imbalance. It often helps if you change your diet to make your body a less appealing host for the organism. Your partner may want to do the same. (Studies suggest that treating the patient's sexual partner may stop recurrence.)

First, try reducing your sugar intake. High-sugar diets stimulate the growth of yeast. Also, add garlic to your diet. A clove once a day is a powerful natural medicine, with specific anti-yeast effects. (That's one segment from a bulb, not the whole thing!) Mash it or chop it fine, mix it with food, and eat it with a meal. Or cut it into chunks and swallow the chunks like pills. Fresh-grown garlic is much better than any garlic supplements. Chew a little parsley afterward if you're concerned about odor, but if you eat garlic regularly and have a good attitude about it, you won't smell of it. Try it, it really works.

Finally, take acidophilus culture. These bacteria are the ones that make milk sour. "Friendly" and natural to the intestinal tract, they may also out-compete yeast in the vaginal area and change the chemistry of the tissues to make them resistant to the fungi. You can buy acidophilus in health food stores, in capsules, or in a milk or carrot-juice base. Check the expiration date to make sure the bacteria are healthy. Take one tablespoon of the liquid culture or one to two of the dry capsules after meals, unless the label directs otherwise.

These changes to your diet may help reverse some of your underlying susceptibility to yeast infections. To treat the infections when they occur, try placing a capsule of acidophilus directly into your vagina once a day, or use a rubber bulb syringe to insert one tablespoon of liquid culture. Another possibility would be tea tree oil, a nontoxic treatment very useful for fungal infections. The oil is extracted from the leaves *of Melaleuca alternifolia.* You can find it in health food or herb stores. Mix $1^1/_2$ tablespoons of the oil in a cup of warm water and use it as a douche once a day. If you experience any irritation, however, discontinue its use.

Resources

Books by Andrew Weil, M.D.

8 Weeks to Optimum Health: A Proven Program for Taking Full Advantage of Your Body's Natural Healing Power. New York: Alfred A. Knopf, 1997.

Spontaneous Healing: How to Discover and Enhance Your Body's Natural Ability to Maintain and Heal Itself. New York: Ballantine Books, 1996.

Natural Health, Natural Medicine: A Comprehensive Manual for Wellness and Self-Care. Rev. ed. Boston: Houghton Mifflin, 1995.

Health and Healing: Understanding Conventional and Alternative Medicine. Rev. ed. Boston: Houghton Mifflin, 1995.

From Chocolate to Morphine: Everything You Need to Know About Mind-Altering Drugs, with Winifred Rosen. Rev. ed. Boston: Houghton Mifflin, 1993.

The Natural Mind: An Investigation of Drugs and the Higher Consciousness. Rev. ed. Boston: Houghton Mifflin, 1986.

The Marriage of the Sun and the Moon: A Quest for Unity in Consciousness. Boston: Houghton Mifflin, 1980.

Other Recommended Books

Lerner, Michael. *Choices in Healing: Integrating the Best of Conventional and Complementary Approaches to Cancer.* Cambridge: MIT Press, 1994.

Reiter, Russel J., and Jo Robinson. *Melatonin: Your Body's Natural Wonder Drug.* New York: Bantam Books, 1995.

Sahelian, Ray, M.D. *DHEA: A Practical Guide.* Garden City Park, New York: Avery Publishing Group, 1996.

Sarno, John, M.D. *Healing Back Pain: The Mind-Body Connection.* New York: Warner Books, 1991.

Other Resources

American Association of Naturopathic Physicians
2366 Eastlake Avenue, Suite 322
Seattle, WA 98102
206 323-7610

American Cancer Society
1599 Clifton Road
Atlanta, GA 30329
800 ACS-2345 (227-2345)

Biofeedback Certification Institute of America
10200 West 44th Avenue, Suite 304
Wheat Ridge, CO 80033
303 420-2902

Home Access
800 HIV TEST (448-8378)

L&H Vitamins
37-10 Crescent Street

Long Island City, NY 11101
800 221-1152

The Vitamin Shoppe
4700 Westside Avenue
North Bergen, NJ 07047
800 223-1216

Program in Integrative Medicine

At the University of Arizona Health Sciences Center,
Tucson, Arizona. For more information, visit the Web
site http://www.ahsc.arizona.edu/integrative_medicine. Or
write: Center for Integrative Medicine, P.O. Box 64089,
Tucson, AZ 85718.

Newsletter

If you would like information on my lectures and infor-
mational products, including my monthly newsletter, *Self
Healing,* please write to: Andrew Weil, M.D., P.O. Box
457, Vail, AZ 85641.

On the Web

"Ask Dr. Weil" answers health questions daily on Time
Warner's Pathfinder Network (www. drweil.com).

Index

About Andrew Weil, M.D.

Dr. Andrew Weil is the leader in the new field of integrative medicine, which combines the best ideas and practices of conventional and alternative medicine. A graduate of Harvard Medical School, he is director of the Program in Integrative Medicine at the University of Arizona, the first program to train physicians in this way at an American medical school. He is also the founder of the Center for Integrative Medicine in Tucson, which is advancing the field worldwide. Dr. Weil is well known as an expert in natural medicine, mind-body interactions, and medical botany, as well as the author of the bestselling *Spontaneous Healing* and *8 Weeks to Optimum Health*. According to Dr. Weil, "Spontaneous healing is not a miracle or a lucky exception, but a fact of biology, the result of the natural healing system that each of us is born with."

About "Ask Dr. Weil"

The "Ask Dr. Weil" program (www.drweil.com) features Andrew Weil, M.D., and is one of the top-rated health sites on the World Wide Web. The recipient of many awards, the "Ask Dr. Weil" program features a daily Q&A with answers to a wide range of health questions, a daily poll, and the Doc Weil Database, which lets readers search hundreds of topics, including material from Dr. Weil's bestselling book *Natural Health, Natural Medicine*. The site also features a Referral Directory (practitioners from acupuncture to Trager work) and DocTalk, a live weekly chat with Dr. Weil. If you have additional questions for Dr. Weil, ask them on his Web site.

About Steven Petrow (Series Editor)

Steven Petrow is the executive producer of the "Ask Dr. Weil" program. Mr. Petrow has held editorial positions with *Life* magazine, *Longevity* magazine, *Fitness*, and *The Wall Street Journal*. He's also been the editor-in-chief of *10 Percent* magazine and *AIDS Digest* and has published five books, including *The HIV Drug Book* and *When Someone You Know Has AIDS*.

Acknowledgments

Richard Pine, Judith Curr, Elisa Wares, and Scott Fagan